Effortless Weight Loss

The Natural Way to a Healthier You; How to shed weight naturally

Daniel. L Wilson

Table of Contents

Introduction

The Benefits of Natural Weight Loss

Losing weight can be a difficult and frustrating journey for many people, with countless fad diets and quick-fix solutions promising instant results. But the truth is, lasting weight loss is about much more than just cutting calories or following a strict meal plan. It's about finding a healthy and sustainable approach to eating, moving, and living that works for you and your body.

This is where natural weight loss comes in. By focusing on nourishing your body with whole, unprocessed foods, incorporating physical activity into your daily routine, and prioritizing self-care practices like sleep and stress management, you can achieve your weight loss goals in a healthy and sustainable way.

But the benefits of natural weight loss extend far beyond just shedding pounds. A healthy lifestyle can also improve your overall well-being, boosting your energy levels, mood, and quality of life. It can even reduce your risk of chronic diseases like heart disease, diabetes, and certain cancers.

In this book, we'll explore the many benefits of natural weight loss and provide you with the tools and strategies you need to succeed on your weight loss journey. From understanding your body's unique needs to overcoming common challenges, we'll help you create a healthy and sustainable plan that works for you.

So let's get started on your journey towards effortless weight loss and a healthier, happier you!

Certainly! Here are a few more points that could be included in the introduction to the book "Effortless Weight Loss: The Natural Way to a Healthier You":

Natural weight loss is all about finding a healthy balance that works for your body and your lifestyle. It's not about deprivation or restriction, but rather about nourishing your body with whole, unprocessed foods and finding joy in movement and self-care practices.

Natural weight loss is a journey, not a destination. It's about making sustainable changes to your habits and lifestyle that you can maintain over the long term. This means finding a balance that works for you, rather than trying to follow a rigid plan that may not be realistic or enjoyable in the long run.

Natural weight loss is about more than just losing weight. It's about improving your overall health and well-being, both physically and mentally. By focusing on nourishing your body, mind, and soul, you can achieve not just a healthy weight, but also increased energy, better sleep, and a greater sense of overall well-being.

The journey towards natural weight loss is unique for each person. There is no one-size-fits-all approach, and what works for one person may not work for another. It's important to find a plan that works for you and your body, and to be kind and compassionate towards yourself as you work towards your goals.

I hope these additional points give you a better understanding of the concept of natural weight loss and the benefits it can bring. Remember, the key is to find a healthy and sustainable approach that works for you, and to focus on nourishing your body, mind, and soul as you work towards your weight loss goals.

Chapter 1

Understanding Your Body and Its Needs

Before you can start on your journey towards natural weight loss, it's important to understand your body and its unique needs. Every person is different, and what works for one person may not work for another. By taking the time to get to know your body, you can create a plan that is tailored to your individual needs and goals.

Here are a few key things to consider when understanding your body and its needs:

Your basal metabolic rate (BMR): Your BMR is the number of calories your body needs to function at rest. It's influenced by factors like your age, gender, weight, and height, and it can help you understand how many calories you need to consume in order to maintain your weight.

Your activity level: Your activity level plays a major role in determining your calorie needs. If you are more active, you will need more calories to fuel your body. On the other hand, if you have a more sedentary lifestyle, you will need fewer calories.

Your body composition: Your body composition refers to the percentage of fat, muscle, and bone in your body. A higher percentage of muscle mass can increase your BMR, as muscle burns more calories than fat.

Your health goals: It's important to consider your overall health goals when creating a natural weight loss plan. Are you looking to lose weight, build muscle, or improve your overall health and well-being? Your goals will help guide your approach to nutrition and physical activity.

By understanding your body and its needs, you can create a natural weight loss plan that is tailored to your individual needs and goals. Remember, the key is to find a healthy and sustainable approach that works for you and your body.

Your body's unique needs can change over time, so it's important to periodically reassess your calorie needs and adjust your plan as needed. For example, if you start an exercise program or experience a significant change in your activity level, your calorie needs may change.

In addition to considering your calorie needs, it's also important to pay attention to the types of nutrients you are consuming. Focus on nourishing your body with a wide variety of whole, unprocessed foods, including plenty of fruits, vegetables, whole grains, and lean proteins.

Don't forget to listen to your body's hunger and fullness cues. Your body is incredibly intelligent and will tell you when it needs nourishment. By learning to tune in to these cues, you can develop a healthy relationship with food and avoid overeating or undereating.

Finally, it's important to remember that weight loss is not the only indicator of health. Your overall well-being is much more than just a number on the scale. By focusing on nourishing your body, mind, and soul, you can achieve a healthy and sustainable weight, as well as increased energy, better sleep, and a greater sense of overall well-being.

I hope these additional points help you better understand the importance of understanding your body and its needs when it comes to natural weight loss. Remember, the key is to find a healthy and sustainable approach that works for you and

your body, and to focus on nourishing
yourself in all aspects of your life.

Chapter 2

The Importance of Mindful Eating

Mindful eating is an important aspect of natural weight loss and overall health. It involves paying attention to your body's hunger and fullness cues, as well as your thoughts, feelings, and experiences around food. By becoming more aware of your eating habits and patterns, you can develop a healthier relationship with food and achieve your weight loss goals in a sustainable way.

Here are a few key principles of mindful eating:

Pay attention to your body's hunger and fullness cues: One of the most important aspects of mindful eating is learning to tune in to your body's hunger and fullness cues. Rather than following a strict meal plan or eating according to the clock, pay attention to your body's natural hunger and fullness signals and stop eating when you feel satisfied.

Slow down and savor your food: Mindful eating involves slowing down and paying attention to the sensory experience of eating. Take the time to chew your food thoroughly, and focus on the flavors, textures, and smells of your food. This can help you enjoy your meals more and feel more satisfied.

Pay attention to your emotions and thoughts around food: Our emotions and thoughts around food can often influence our eating habits. By becoming more aware of these emotions and thoughts, you can identify any unhealthy patterns and develop healthier coping strategies.

Practice gratitude: One of the key principles of mindful eating is gratitude. Take the time to appreciate the food you are eating, and

recognize the effort and resources that went
into producing it.

Don't use food as a reward or punishment.
Food should be enjoyed, not used as a
reward or punishment. Avoid using food as
a way to cope with emotions or stress, and
instead focus on finding healthy ways to
manage your emotions.

Remember that it's okay to indulge every
once in a while. While it's important to focus
on nourishing your body with healthy foods,
it's also okay to indulge in your favorite
treats every once in a while. The key is to do
so mindfully and in moderation, rather than
restricting yourself and then overindulging.

Be mindful of portion sizes. It's important to
pay attention to portion sizes, especially if
you are trying to lose weight. Use portion
control tools like measuring cups and
spoons or smaller plates to help you get a
sense of appropriate portion sizes.

Don't be afraid to seek help if you are struggling with disordered eating. If you are struggling with disordered eating or have a difficult time following mindful eating practices, it may be helpful to seek the guidance of a healthcare professional or a registered dietitian. They can provide support and guidance to help you develop a healthy relationship with food.

By eating mindfully, you can develop a healthy and sustainable approach to eating that supports your weight loss goals.

Chapter 3

Incorporating Physical Activity into Your Life

Physical activity is an important aspect of natural weight loss and overall health. Regular physical activity can help you lose weight, build muscle, improve your cardiovascular health, and increase your energy levels. It can also improve your mood and reduce your risk of chronic diseases like heart disease, diabetes, and certain cancers.

But finding the right type of physical activity for you can be a challenge. With so many options to choose from, it's important to find something that you enjoy and that fits into your lifestyle. Here are a few tips for incorporating physical activity into your life:

Find activities you enjoy: The best physical activity is the one that you enjoy and will be consistent with. This could be anything from walking, running, or cycling to dancing, yoga, or team sports. By finding activities that you enjoy, you'll be more likely to stick with them in the long run.

Make it a habit: Incorporating physical activity into your daily routine can help you stay consistent and motivated. Try to make physical activity a habit by scheduling it at the same time each day or week. You might also try finding a workout buddy or joining a group fitness class to stay motivated.

Mix it up: Mixing up your physical activity can help keep things interesting and prevent boredom. Try incorporating a variety of activities into your routine, such as cardio, strength training, and flexibility work.

Be realistic: It's important to be realistic about what you can fit into your schedule and what your body can handle. Don't try to do too much too soon, as this can lead to burnout and injury. Instead, start slowly and gradually increase your intensity and duration as you become more comfortable and fit.

By incorporating physical activity into your life in a way that works for you, you can improve your health, boost your energy levels, and support your natural weight loss journey. Remember to listen to your body and make adjustments as needed, and to always prioritize safety and injury prevention.

Don't forget about the importance of rest and recovery. Physical activity can be beneficial for your health, but it's important to allow your body time to rest and recover between workouts. This can help prevent injury and allow your muscles to repair and grow stronger.

It's okay to start small and work your way up. If you're new to exercise or haven't been active in a while, it's okay to start small and gradually increase your intensity and duration over time. Even just a few minutes of physical activity each day can have significant health benefits.

Don't be afraid to try new things. Keep an open mind and be willing to try new activities or sports. You never know what you might enjoy until you try it.

Don't get discouraged if you have setbacks. It's normal to have off days or to experience setbacks, and it's important to be kind to yourself and not get discouraged. Remember that physical activity is a journey and that it's okay to take breaks or adjust your plan as needed.

I hope these additional points help you better understand the importance of incorporating physical activity into your life as a part of a natural weight loss journey.

Chapter 4

The Role of Sleep in Weight Loss

Getting enough sleep is an important aspect of natural weight loss and overall health. Not only does sleep help you feel rested and refreshed, but it also plays a crucial role in regulating your appetite and metabolism.

Here are a few ways that sleep impacts weight loss:

Sleep affects hunger hormones: Sleep deprivation can disrupt the balance of two hormones that regulate appetite: ghrelin and leptin. Ghrelin, a hormone produced in the stomach, increases hunger and appetite, while leptin, a hormone produced in fat cells, reduces hunger and increases feelings of fullness. When you don't get enough sleep, your body produces more ghrelin and less leptin, leading to increased hunger and cravings.

Sleep impacts metabolism: Adequate sleep is important for maintaining a healthy metabolism. Studies have shown that people who don't get enough sleep tend to have a slower metabolism and may be more likely to gain weight. On the other hand, getting enough sleep can help boost your metabolism and support weight loss.

Sleep affects physical activity: Lack of sleep can also impact your energy levels and motivation to be physically active. When you're feeling tired and sluggish, it can be harder to find the energy and motivation to exercise. On the other hand, getting enough sleep can help you feel more energetic and motivated to move.

It's important to prioritize getting enough sleep as a part of your natural weight loss journey. Aim for 7-9 hours of sleep per night, and create a sleep-friendly environment by keeping your bedroom dark, quiet, and cool. Avoid screens and caffeine before bed, and try incorporating relaxation techniques like meditation or deep breathing to help you wind down.

By prioritizing sleep, you can support your weight loss efforts and improve your overall health and well-being.

Sleep affects cognitive function and decision-making. Lack of sleep can impair your ability to think clearly and make good decisions, which can lead to poor food choices and less self-control. On the other hand, getting enough sleep can help improve your cognitive function and decision-making skills, making it easier to resist temptations and make healthy choices.

The quality of your sleep is just as important as the quantity. It's not just about how many hours you sleep, but also about the quality of that sleep. Make sure you are getting

deep, restful sleep by following good sleep
hygiene practices, such as avoiding screens
and caffeine before bed, creating a relaxing
sleep environment, and establishing a
consistent bedtime routine.

Chronic sleep deprivation can have serious
health consequences. In addition to
impacting weight loss, chronic sleep
deprivation has been linked to a range of
health problems, including an increased risk
of heart disease, diabetes, and certain
cancers. It can also impact your mood,
energy levels, and overall well-being.

Sleep can be affected by other factors, such
as stress and diet. Stress and unhealthy
eating habits can both impact your sleep
quality. It's important to address these
factors as a part of your natural weight loss
journey, in order to support healthy sleep
habits.

Don't be afraid to seek help if you are having trouble sleeping. If you are consistently having trouble falling asleep or staying asleep, it may be worth speaking with a healthcare professional. They can help identify any underlying causes and provide strategies for improving your sleep quality.

 Remember, it's important to prioritize getting enough quality sleep as a part of your weight loss journey, and to address any sleep issues that may arise.

Chapter 5

Stress Management for Sustainable Weight Loss

Stress management is an important aspect of natural weight loss and overall health. Chronic stress can have a negative impact on your physical and mental well-being, and it can also disrupt your eating habits and weight loss efforts. By learning to manage stress effectively, you can support your weight loss goals and improve your overall health and well-being.

Here are a few tips for managing stress as a part of your natural weight loss journey:

Practice relaxation techniques: Relaxation techniques like deep breathing, meditation, or yoga can help you reduce stress and improve your overall well-being. These techniques can be practiced anytime, anywhere, and can help you feel more calm and centered.

Exercise regularly: Physical activity is a great way to reduce stress and improve your overall health. It can help boost your mood, reduce anxiety, and improve your sleep quality.

Eat a healthy, balanced diet: A healthy, balanced diet can help support your physical and mental well-being and reduce stress. Focus on nourishing your body with a variety of whole, unprocessed foods, and avoid relying on unhealthy coping mechanisms like comfort eating or binging.

Get enough sleep: Adequate sleep is essential for managing stress and supporting your overall health. Aim for 7-9 hours of sleep per night, and create a sleep-friendly environment by keeping your bedroom dark, quiet, and cool.

By incorporating these stress management strategies into your natural weight loss journey, you can improve your overall health and well-being and better support your weight loss efforts. Remember, it's important to find a balance that works for you and your body, and to be kind and compassionate towards yourself as you work towards your goals.

Here are few points:

Identify your stress triggers: One of the first steps in managing stress is identifying what triggers it. Take the time to reflect on what causes you stress and try to find ways to minimize or avoid those triggers.

Seek support: Don't be afraid to seek support when you're feeling overwhelmed. Talk to a trusted friend or family member, or consider working with a therapist or counselor.

Practice self-care: Taking care of yourself is an important aspect of stress management. Make sure to set aside time for self-care activities like exercise, meditation, or hobbies that you enjoy.

Find healthy ways to cope: It's normal to turn to food or other unhealthy coping mechanisms when you're feeling stressed, but it's important to find healthier ways to cope. Try practicing relaxation techniques, talking to someone, or finding a physical outlet for your stress, like going for a walk or hitting the gym.

Remember that it's okay to take breaks: It's important to remember that it's okay to take breaks and slow down when you're feeling overwhelmed. Don't be afraid to take time for yourself and prioritize your well-being.

Chapter 6

The Power of a Plant-Based Diet

A plant-based diet is a type of diet that emphasizes whole, unprocessed plant foods, such as fruits, vegetables, whole grains, legumes, nuts, and seeds. Plant-based diets can be a powerful tool for natural weight loss and overall health, as they are rich in nutrients, fiber, and antioxidants and can help support healthy digestion, metabolism, and overall well-being.

Here are a few key benefits of a plant-based diet for weight loss and overall health:

Weight loss: Plant-based diets have been shown to be effective for weight loss. They are often lower in calories and fat than diets that include animal products, and they can help you feel fuller and more satisfied due to their high fiber content.

Improved digestion: Plant-based diets are rich in fiber, which can help support healthy digestion and prevent constipation. They can also promote the growth of beneficial bacteria in the gut, which can support overall health.

Lower risk of chronic diseases: Plant-based diets have been linked to a lower risk of chronic diseases, such as heart disease, diabetes, and certain cancers. They are also associated with a lower risk of obesity and other weight-related conditions.

Environmental sustainability: In addition to the health benefits, a plant-based diet can also have a positive impact on the environment. Plant-based foods tend to have a lower carbon footprint than animal-based foods, and they can help reduce water and land use.

Versatility: Plant-based diets can be incredibly versatile and can include a wide variety of foods. There are many plant-based protein sources, such as beans, lentils, tofu, and nuts, as well as a wide range of fruits, vegetables, whole grains, and healthy fats.

Customizability: A plant-based diet can be tailored to meet your individual needs and preferences. You can choose to follow a vegan diet, which excludes all animal products, or a vegetarian diet, which includes some animal products, such as eggs and dairy. You can also choose to follow a whole food plant-based diet, which emphasizes whole, unprocessed plant foods, or a more flexible plant-based diet that includes some processed or refined foods.

Support and resources: There are many resources available to help you get started on a plant-based diet, including recipe books, blogs, and online communities. You can also speak with a healthcare professional or a registered dietitian for personalized support and guidance.

Remember, the key is to find a plant-based approach that works for you and your body, and to focus on nourishing yourself with a variety of whole, unprocessed plant foods.

Chapter 7

Creative Ways to Stay Motivated on Your Weight Loss Journey

Staying motivated on your weight loss journey can be a challenge, but it's an important factor in achieving your goals. By finding creative ways to stay motivated, you can stay on track and make progress towards your goals.

Here are a few tips for staying motivated on your weight loss journey:

Set achievable goals: Setting realistic and achievable goals can help you stay motivated and on track. Rather than trying to achieve unrealistic goals, focus on setting small, achievable goals that you can work towards consistently.

Find a support system: Having a support system of friends, family, or a healthcare professional can be a powerful source of motivation. Consider joining a weight loss group or finding a workout buddy to help keep you accountable and motivated.

Celebrate your progress: It's important to recognize and celebrate your progress, no matter how small. This can help boost your motivation and confidence, and keep you motivated to continue on your journey.

Find activities you enjoy: Incorporating physical activity into your weight loss journey can be a great source of motivation. But it's important to find activities that you enjoy, so that you're more likely to stick with them in the long run.

Stay positive: It's normal to have setbacks and challenges on your weight loss journey, but it's important to stay positive and focus on the progress you've made.

Certainly! Here are a few more points that could be included in Chapter 7, "Creative Ways to Stay Motivated on Your Weight Loss Journey," for the book "Effortless Weight Loss: The Natural Way to a Healthier You":

Make a plan: Having a clear plan can help keep you on track and motivated. Consider creating a detailed meal plan, setting specific exercise goals, or scheduling regular check-ins with a healthcare professional or coach.

Find accountability: Having someone to hold you accountable can be a powerful source of motivation. Consider working with a coach or personal trainer, or finding an accountability partner or group to help keep you on track.

Keep a journal: Writing down your progress and thoughts can be a great way to stay motivated and track your progress. Consider keeping a food and exercise journal, or writing down your goals and achievements.

Get enough sleep: Adequate sleep is essential for maintaining energy and motivation. Make sure to prioritize getting enough sleep as a part of your weight loss journey, and create a sleep-friendly environment by keeping your bedroom dark, quiet, and cool.

Seek professional help if needed: If you are struggling to stay motivated or are experiencing negative thoughts or feelings around your weight loss journey, it may be worth seeking professional help. A healthcare professional or therapist can help you address any underlying issues and provide strategies for staying motivated and on track.

I hope these additional points help you better understand the importance of staying motivated on your weight loss journey and

provide some creative ideas for how to do
so. Remember, it's important to find what
works for you and your body, and to be kind
and compassionate towards yourself as you
work towards your goals.

Chapter 8

Overcoming Common Challenges in Natural Weight Loss

Natural weight loss can be a journey that involves ups and downs, and it's normal to face challenges along the way. By learning how to overcome these challenges, you can stay on track and make progress towards your goals.

Here are a few common challenges in natural weight loss, and some tips for how to overcome them:

Difficulty sticking to a healthy diet: One of the most common challenges in weight loss is sticking to a healthy diet. To overcome this challenge, try planning ahead and preparing healthy meals and snacks in advance, so that you have healthy options on hand when you're feeling hungry. It can also be helpful to keep unhealthy foods out of the house, or to have healthier alternatives available.

Lack of motivation: It's normal to feel unmotivated at times, especially when you're making lifestyle changes. To overcome this challenge, try finding activities that you enjoy, setting achievable goals, and celebrating your progress. It can also be helpful to seek support from friends, family, or a healthcare professional.

Difficulty with physical activity: Incorporating physical activity into your weight loss journey can be a challenge, especially if you're not used to being active. To overcome this challenge, try starting small and gradually increasing your activity level. Find activities that you enjoy, and try to make exercise a regular part of your routine.

Emotional eating: Emotional eating, or eating in response to emotions rather than hunger, can be a common challenge in weight loss. To overcome this challenge, try identifying the emotions and triggers that lead to emotional eating, and develop healthy coping strategies to address those emotions. This could involve practicing relaxation techniques.

Here are a few more points that could be included in Chapter 8, "Overcoming Common Challenges in Natural Weight Loss,"

Time constraints: Managing a busy schedule can be a challenge when it comes to natural weight loss. To overcome this challenge, try setting aside specific times for healthy meals and physical activity, and make the most of your time by preparing healthy meals in advance and finding ways to incorporate activity into your daily routine.

Social pressures: It can be difficult to stick to a healthy lifestyle when you're surrounded by unhealthy habits or social pressure to eat or drink unhealthy foods. To overcome this challenge, try finding supportive friends and family members who can help you stay on track, and remind yourself of your reasons for pursuing natural weight loss.

Hormonal imbalances: Hormonal imbalances can sometimes be a factor in weight gain or difficulty losing weight. If you suspect that hormonal imbalances may be contributing to your weight loss challenges, it may be worth speaking with a healthcare professional to explore potential underlying causes and treatment options.

Medical conditions: In some cases, weight loss challenges may be related to underlying medical conditions, such as thyroid issues or insulin resistance. If you are experiencing difficulty losing weight or are experiencing other unusual symptoms, it's important to speak with a healthcare professional to explore potential underlying causes and treatment options.

Chapter 9

Celebrating Your Success and Maintaining Your Weight Loss

Congratulations on your weight loss success! It's a big accomplishment and something to be celebrated. Here are some tips for celebrating your success and maintaining your weight loss:

Reflect on your journey: Take some time to reflect on the hard work and dedication it took to get to this point. Consider keeping a journal to document your progress and the changes you've made to your lifestyle.

Celebrate with non-food related activities: It's important to find ways to celebrate your success that don't involve food. This can help you avoid falling back into old habits or overeating. Consider doing something active like going for a hike or trying a new workout class. Or, do something relaxing like getting a massage or going to a movie.

Don't be too hard on yourself: It's normal to have setbacks or slip-ups along the way. If you do have a less healthy meal or miss a workout, try not to beat yourself up over it. Instead, focus on getting back on track and moving forward.

Keep up the healthy habits: Maintaining your weight loss means continuing to make healthy choices. This includes eating a balanced diet, getting regular exercise, and finding ways to manage stress. Don't be afraid to seek support from friends, family, or a healthcare professional if you need help staying on track.

Treat yourself occasionally: It's okay to indulge in your favorite foods or treats every once in a while, as long as it's in moderation. Just be sure to balance it out with healthy eating and physical activity.

Remember, weight loss is a journey, and it's important to celebrate your successes along the way. By continuing to make healthy choices and finding ways to celebrate your progress, you can maintain your weight loss and live a healthy, balanced lifestyle.

Here are some additional tips for celebrating your weight loss success and maintaining your progress:

Set new goals: Reaching your weight loss goal is a great accomplishment, but it's important to continue setting and working towards new goals. This can help keep you motivated and focused on your health and wellness journey. Consider setting goals related to exercise, nutrition, or self-care.

Find a support system: Surround yourself with people who support and encourage your healthy habits. This can be friends, family, or a support group. Having a strong support system can help you stay motivated and on track.

Stay positive: It's important to maintain a positive mindset on your weight loss journey. This can help you stay motivated and focused on your goals. Try to find the silver lining in any setbacks or challenges you face and remember to be kind to yourself.

Stay active: Regular physical activity is an important part of maintaining your weight loss. Find activities that you enjoy and make them a regular part of your routine. This can be anything from a structured exercise class to a leisurely walk in nature.

Find healthy ways to cope with stress: Stress can be a major factor in weight gain or weight loss. When you're feeling stressed, it's important to find healthy ways to cope with it. This can include activities like yoga, meditation, or exercise. It's also important to prioritize self-care and find ways to relax and unwind.

Maintaining your weight loss takes effort and dedication, but it's worth it for the improved health and quality of life it can bring. By setting goals, finding a support system, staying active, and finding healthy ways to cope with stress, you can succeed in maintaining your weight loss and living a healthy, balanced lifestyle.